Cold Therapy

A Beginner's 5-Step Guide on Getting Started with Cryotherapy for Pain Relief, Depression, and Other Use Cases

FELICITY PAULMAN

Introduction

There are a wide variety of approaches to choose from when it comes to the management of pain. Some people get comfort from drugs, while others favor more natural approaches such as chiropractic care or acupuncture. Acupuncture and chiropractic care are two examples.

Cold therapy is a potentially useful choice for patients who choose a treatment that requires more active participation from them. This treatment, which is often referred to as cryotherapy, involves subjecting the body to exceedingly low temperatures. This can be accomplished with the use of ice packs, immersion in cold water, or even nitrogen gas.

It is believed that cold treatment works by numbing the nerve endings and lowering inflammation, however the specific mechanism that causes these effects is not entirely known. In addition to this, there is evidence from certain studies that shows it may also aid to strengthen the immune system.

Although further research is required to verify these advantages, cold therapy is a risk-free and non-invasive treatment option that has the potential to assist patients who suffer from chronic pain with some respite.

In this introduction to cold treatment, often known as cryotherapy, we are going to look at the following specific areas:

- What is cold therapy?
- History of cold therapy
- Cold therapy techniques
- How does cold therapy work?
- Benefits of cold therapy
- Use cases of cold therapy
- A potential 5-step guide on how to get started with cold therapy
- Heat therapy vs. cold therapy
- Risks or potential side effects of cold therapy
- Who should not use cold therapy

If you want to know more about cold therapy and how to get started, read on!

Table of Contents

WHAT IS COLD THERAPY?

Cryotherapy, which is more often referred to as cold therapy, is a treatment that involves the use of extremely low temperatures to alleviate pain and promote healing. Some people believe that using cold treatment can help reduce inflammation, speed up the healing process, and enhance blood circulation. These are all claims that are made by proponents of using cold therapy.

Even though there is some evidence from scientific studies to back up these claims, further study is required to verify that cold treatment is effective. At the moment, the application of cold therapy is most frequently utilized in the treatment of soft tissue injuries such as sprains and bruises. Additionally, it may be utilized to alleviate the pain that is brought on by disorders like migraines, fibromyalgia, and arthritis.

When used appropriately, cold treatment is usually considered to be safe and well-accepted by patients. On the other hand, it is essential to prevent freezing the skin, as this might harm the surrounding tissue. Before beginning cold treatment, those who are pregnant or who suffer from specific medical disorders should consult with a physician.

HISTORY OF COLD THERAPY

Hippocrates, who lived in ancient Greece, was a proponent of using cold to treat a range of ailments, including fever. The use of cold in ancient medicine stretches back to the time of Hippocrates. In the ensuing years, throughout the 18th and 19th centuries, medical practitioners in Europe adopted the concept of employing cold as a therapy for many illnesses.

During this period, the practice of taking a cold bath was widely considered to be a useful type of medical therapy due to the belief that these baths might reduce inflammation and activate the immune system of the body. The medical profession in America eventually came around to the idea of taking cold baths, but for many years afterward, there was much controversy regarding the practice's effectiveness. Although some people were under the impression that cold treatment may alleviate pain and inflammation, others refused to believe it.

After the turn of the 20th century, scientific evidence came to be acknowledged that demonstrated the usefulness of cold therapy. Research shows that chilling the body can reduce inflammation, increase recovery time, and assist treat a variety of medical ailments, but the practice of taking a bath in cold water is still debated today as a method of treatment.

The treatment of musculoskeletal injuries with cold therapy is currently the most popular practice. Additionally, it may be utilized to alleviate the pain that is brought on by chronic ailments such as migraines, arthritis, and fibromyalgia, amongst others.

COLD THERAPY TECHNIQUES

A wide range of ailments can be helped by employing several cold treatment procedures in a variety of different ways. Because every approach comes with a unique set of advantages and disadvantages, it is essential to have a conversation with a medical professional about the available choices before beginning any kind of therapy.

Ice Packs: The use of ice packs is one of the cold treatment methods that is used the most frequently. Ice packs, which can be found for sale in the majority of pharmacies and drugstores, can be utilized to alleviate symptoms such as pain, swelling, and inflammation. Ice packs should be applied to the afflicted region for a period of fifteen to twenty minutes at a time, and the treatment can be repeated multiple times a day.

Cryotherapy: Cryotherapy is a type of cold treatment that involves the use of temperatures that are extremely low to cure a variety of painful conditions and inflammation. Cryotherapy can be carried out in several different methods, such as whole-body cryotherapy (WBC), targeted cryotherapy, and chambers specifically designed for cryotherapy. Localized cryotherapy is when extremely low temperatures are applied to a specific area of the body, whereas whole-body cryotherapy (WBC) entails standing within an enclosed chamber that is filled with extremely cold air for two to three minutes.

Cold Compresses: Cold compresses are another prominent technique used in cold therapy that may be utilized to assist in the reduction of pain and inflammation. It is possible to make cold compresses by first soaking a clean cloth in cold water and then applying it to the region that is hurt for 10 to 15 minutes. Additionally, cold compresses are available for purchase at the majority of pharmacies and drugstores.

Immersion in Cold Water: Another kind of cold treatment is known as cold water immersion, which includes submerging one's entire body in cold water for some time. An immersion in cold water can be accomplished in a variety of ways, such as by utilizing an ice bath, taking a cold shower or bath, swimming in a cold pool, or swimming in an ice bath. The length of time spent immersed in the water will differ from person to person according to how well they can withstand the cold.

Ice Massage: Ice massage is a form of cold treatment that involves rubbing the afflicted region with an ice cube for a period of five to ten minutes at a time. Ice massage can be performed many times per day. The ice massage treatment can be repeated as many times per day as necessary. To avoid getting frostbite, it is essential to make sure that the ice cube is protected by a thin towel or piece of fabric.

Coolant spray: Isopentane and menthol are the active components of a cooling spray, which also contains other chemicals. Isopentane functions as a propellant, accelerating the pace at which the liquid evaporates. Menthol is a naturally occurring chemical molecule that may be used to bring a refreshing sensation to the skin. Isopentane and menthol, when combined, produce a sense of coolness that, when combined, can help relieve pain.

The use of coolant spray is a common treatment for aching muscles, as well as arthritis and headaches. Inflammation and edema are both conditions that might benefit from its usage. The Coolant spray is sprayed topically on the injured region, and the normal duration of its pain-relieving effects is around half an hour. The spray can be reapplied as often as necessary, and its usage is generally considered to be risk-free for the vast majority of people.

Cold Lasers: Cold lasers are a sort of low-level laser treatment that helps relieve pain and inflammation by making use of low levels of light. Cold lasers are also known as ice lasers. The use of cold lasers is normally limited to brief intervals (ranging from five to ten minutes) and may be repeated multiple times daily, depending on the requirements.

Cold Therapy Machines: People searching for pain relief are turning more and more frequently to cold therapy machines as an option. The devices alleviate pain by moving cold water via pads or wraps that are applied to the part of the body that is hurting and then circulating the water there. As a result of the water's cool temperature, inflammation is reduced, and the affected region is rendered numb, which provides relief from both acute and chronic pain.

Since there is a wide variety of cold treatment equipment available on the market, it is essential to pick the device that is most suited to meet your requirements. While some devices are built specifically for use in clinical or hospital settings, others are designed to be portable enough to be utilized in the comfort of one's own home.

Pads and wraps are also available in a wide variety of sizes and forms, allowing you to select an option that is an excellent match for your particular form. Cold therapy machines are becoming an increasingly popular choice for those who are searching for an alternative to the use of medicine to alleviate pain. These machines can give a solution to gain relief from pain that is both safe and effective.

HOW DOES COLD THERAPY WORK?

Cryotherapy, which is more often referred to as cold therapy, is a form of medical treatment that makes use of temperatures that are very low to alleviate pain and swelling. The number of individuals who are interested in complementary and alternative methods of treatment has increased over the past several decades, which has contributed to a rise in the usage of this treatment method for a wide range of conditions. So, how exactly does treatment of this kind take place?

Inflammation, swelling, and even bruising can occur after an injury has been sustained by a person. All of these things are a part of the natural healing process that occurs within the body, such as an increase in blood flow to the region to assist with the repair. Sadly, the culmination of all of these factors can sometimes result in suffering.

The nerves are dulled and inflammation is decreased by the use of cold treatment. The veins in the skin around an injury will become more constricted if the surrounding region is cold. This decreases the amount of blood that flows to the region, which in turn lessens the swelling and discomfort. The decreased blood flow also helps to numb the nerves, which further reduces the amount of pain that is experienced. In addition, the cool temperature can assist in the reduction of inflammation by lowering the metabolic rate of the cells that are responsible for the condition.

The use of cold therapy is a fantastic method for alleviating pain and suffering, and it also has the potential to assist speed up the healing process. Although it is vital to get medical assistance if you are having severe or ongoing pain, cold therapy can give some much-needed relief in many circumstances. If you are experiencing severe or ongoing pain, it is necessary to seek medical attention.

BENEFITS OF COLD THERAPY

When it comes to making a full recovery after an injury, a lot of individuals have the misconception that the more time they put in at the gym or physical therapy, the better it will be for them. What if, on the other hand, there was a more straightforward approach to hasten the recovery process? It has come to light that there is, and participation in a cold treatment program is required. It's a common misconception that the only people who can benefit from cold treatment are athletes who have just experienced an acute injury. People living normal lives who want to enhance their general health and sense of well-being can also make use of it as a tool to help them do so.

The following is a list of some of the potential benefits that cold treatment can offer:

Reduces Inflammation: One of the most important advantages of cold treatment is that it may assist in bringing about a reduction in the level of inflammation that is present. When the body is attempting to recover after an accident or an illness, one of the normal processes that take place is inflammation. Chronic inflammation, on the other hand, can result in a wide range of health complications, including coronary heart disease, arthritis, and diabetes. The use of cold therapy can be beneficial in the treatment of inflammation because it can assist to constrict blood vessels and reduce swelling.

Pain Relief: Cold treatment is another method that is useful in alleviating pain. This is because exposure to low temperatures helps to numb nerve endings, which in turn helps to limit the number of pain signals that are transmitted to the brain. A common treatment for the discomfort caused by injuries such as muscle sprains and strains is the application of cold compresses. It has also been shown to be effective in the treatment of painful illnesses such as migraines and arthritis.

Increases Blood Flow: Cold treatment has been shown to increase blood flow, which is another benefit. Inadequate circulation can be the root cause of several health issues, including tiredness, joint discomfort, and numbness in the hands and feet. The constriction of blood vessels and the subsequent increase in blood flow are two beneficial side effects of cold treatment for improving circulation. This can assist the cells and tissues in the body receive more oxygen and nutrients than they would otherwise receive.

Increased White Blood Cell Production: Cold treatment can also assist to increase white blood cell production, which is beneficial for increasing one's immunity. White blood cells are the cells in the blood that are in charge of fighting off infections and diseases. The body begins a process known as thermogenesis when it is subjected to cold temperatures. This process contributes to an increase in the production of white blood cells and helps the body fight against infections.

Reduces Cellulite: Cellulite is a specific sort of fat that has the propensity to gather in the area of the thighs, buttocks, and stomach. Cellulite may be reduced. It is frequently characterized as having the look of an "orange peel" or "dimpled" surface. Cellulite does not pose any threat to a person's health; yet, many individuals find it to be visually unpleasant. Cellulite can be reduced with the use of cold treatment by triggering the breakdown of fat cells and enhancing circulation.

Relieves Depression: Cold therapy can also be good in treating depression, making it a potentially useful treatment option. Researchers have discovered that being exposed to cold temperatures can help the body produce more serotonin and dopamine, which are both neurotransmitters that play a role in the regulation of mood. In addition, there is evidence that cold treatment might lower stress levels, which is another factor that can contribute to an improvement in mood.

These are just some of the many advantages that may be gained from undergoing cold treatment. It has the potential to be an efficient instrument for alleviating pain, lowering inflammation, and enhancing immune function.

In addition to this, it has the potential to enhance circulation and lessen the appearance of cellulite. Last but not least, it is useful in the treatment of depression by elevating levels of both serotonin and dopamine. Because it has the potential to provide so many advantages, there is no reason to avoid trying cold therapy.

USE CASES OF COLD THERAPY

The use of extremely cold temperatures sometimes referred to as cryotherapy can be used to treat a wide range of medical disorders. Cold therapy may be used to treat a broad variety of illnesses, even though sports medicine and physical therapy are the fields in which it is most widely utilized. Here are ten different applications of cold treatment.

Sore muscles: Inflamed and painful muscles can benefit from the use of cold therapy since it helps to constrict blood vessels, which in turn lowers swelling and inflammation. Additionally, it may aid to numb the region and provide pain relief. The use of cold treatment is usual for providing comfort for a shorter period, and it is not indicated for pain that is persistent. On the other hand, people who only suffer occasional muscular soreness may find that applying ice to the affected area is an excellent technique to lessen the discomfort and speed up the recovery process.

Inflammation: Inflammation is a normal reaction of the body to injury or infection; but, when it becomes chronic, it can lead to a wide range of health issues. Inflammation can be caused by: Cryotherapy, often known as cold therapy, which is a form of treatment that includes subjecting the body to extremely low temperatures. This can help to relieve inflammation by narrowing blood vessels and bringing down swelling in the affected area. Cryotherapy is a successful treatment for a wide range of inflammatory disorders, including tendinitis, arthritis, and carpal tunnel syndrome, among others.

Arthritis: Arthritis is a disorder that affects a large number of people and is characterized by pain and stiffness in the joints. It is noticed more frequently in persons who are middle-aged or older, although it can also affect younger people. Because arthritis causes inflammation, treatment with a cold can help to alleviate some of the associated symptoms, including pain and stiffness. The reduced swelling and numbness in the nerves are both benefits of the cool temperature. Additionally, it may assist in improving circulation and alleviating muscular spasms.

Fibromyalgia: People who suffer from fibromyalgia may find that cold therapy is a helpful treatment option for their condition. The widespread pain, exhaustion, and other symptoms that are associated with fibromyalgia are caused by the disorder known as fibromyalgia. These symptoms can be alleviated with the use of cold treatment, which works by lowering inflammation and dulling pain. There are a few different approaches to cold treatment, the most common of which include the use of ice packs, cold showers, and cryotherapy.

However, it is essential to make prudent use of cold treatment because it also has the potential to make some symptoms worse. For instance, persons who suffer from fibromyalgia frequently have sensitive skin; therefore, they must avoid coming into direct contact with the ice to prevent frostbite.

In addition, people who have fibromyalgia frequently struggle to maintain a normal body temperature, which is why it is essential to begin exposure to cold temperatures with just short bursts of time and progressively lengthen the time spent in the cold as tolerated. The proper application of cold treatment can be an effective strategy for the management of the symptoms of fibromyalgia when utilized as intended.

Migraines: People who suffer from migraines are all too familiar with the excruciating agony that frequently accompanies these severe headaches. Even while there is a wide selection of drugs that can assist alleviate the pain, the most effective treatments are not always the ones that are the most complicated.

One of these treatments is to apply ice to the affected area, which has been shown to help constrict blood vessels and decrease inflammation. One method for accomplishing this is to make use of a cold compress or ice pack or even to take a cold shower. Even while the comfort may not come immediately, it may still be able to give some much-needed respite from the throbbing agony that is associated with migraines.

Fever: Fever is a symptom that the body is fighting off an infection, and the level of the fever can range from being somewhat unpleasant to life-threatening. Fever is a sign that the body is fighting off an infection. The production of perspiration and overall cooling of the body are the two primary mechanisms by which a fever can be brought under control.

However, because these therapies might cause the body to lose heat more rapidly than normal, it is essential to exercise extreme caution when utilizing them. If the fever does not respond to therapy or if it is accompanied by other symptoms, such as severe bodily pains or trouble breathing, it is essential to seek medical help as soon as possible. People may assist guarantee that they are safe and comfortable while their bodies fight off illness if they are aware of how to treat a fever. This knowledge can be used to treat fevers.

Sunburn: Applying ice to a sunburn can help alleviate the discomfort and lessen the swelling that results from the burn. Sunburn is a sort of radiation damage that can occur to the skin when it is subjected to the sun's ultraviolet (UV) rays for an extended period. Exposure to UV radiation will result in the skin becoming red and becoming irritated.

The discomfort and swelling associated with a sunburn can be alleviated by applying cold compresses to the affected area. Wrapping an ice pack in a towel and applying it to the afflicted region for ten to fifteen minutes at a time is the most effective approach to providing cold therapy. You may also try taking a shower or bath in cool water to assist ease the discomfort and swelling in your body.

Bites from insects: Applying ice to bites might help decrease swelling and discomfort associated with the bite. The region becomes numb as a result of the freezing temperature, and the constriction of blood vessels contributes to a reduction in inflammation. To avoid causing harm to the tissues, it is essential to limit the duration of each cold to no more than 10 minutes. It is possible to shield the skin from the cold by using a bag of frozen veggies or wrapping ice in a towel first.

Skin conditions: Cold therapy has been used for a long time to treat a variety of conditions, both medical and cosmetic. It is commonly used to treat skin conditions. When the skin is subjected to extremely cold temperatures, the blood vessels in the skin constrict, which in turn reduces inflammation.

Psoriasis, eczema, and acne are just some of the conditions that can benefit from this treatment. The usage of cold treatment is another method that may be utilized to enhance the look of the skin. A more youthful appearance can be achieved by minimizing the appearance of redness and puffiness on the skin.

Recovery following surgery: Cold therapy is frequently used as a treatment for injuries because of its ability to assist in reducing swelling and discomfort. Additionally, it can enhance circulation, which in turn speeds up the healing process. The process of recovery after surgery is a lengthy and challenging endeavor; however, cold treatment can assist to make the process a little bit simpler. Cold treatment can assist patients in recovering more rapidly and with less discomfort. It does this by lowering swelling and pain, boosting circulation, and accelerating the body's natural healing process.

The application of cold to the affected area is a flexible treatment that may be used to address a wide range of medical issues. If you need pain relief, relief from inflammation, or treatment for a skin problem, you should think about utilizing cryotherapy.

A POTENTIAL 5-STEP PLAN ON HOW TO GET STARTED

If you are thinking about trying cold treatment, the following information might serve as a starting point for you.

1. Step 1: Determine When to Use Cold Therapy

Cold therapy is an effective treatment for a wide range of illnesses, including those listed below. In most cases, it is used for the treatment of acute ailments like sprains and strains. Chronic pain, arthritis, migraines, and headaches are some other conditions that may benefit from their use. On the other hand, if you have an open wound or difficulties with your circulation, you should not utilize cold treatment. Before commencing any treatment, you should always discuss your options with a trained medical expert, especially if you are unclear about whether or not cold therapy is appropriate for you.

2. Step 2: Select the Mode of Cold Therapy That Best Suits You

Selecting the cold treatment approach that best suits your needs is the second step in getting started with cold therapy. The use of ice packs is the most frequent way, but you may also use cold gel packs, frozen peas, or ice water baths. Ice packs are the most common option. Cryotherapy chambers and cold compression wraps are two other ways that cold treatment can be administered.

Before making a decision, you need to weigh the benefits of each approach against the drawbacks associated with using that approach. For instance, ice packs are simple to employ but have the potential to be unpleasant and aggravate skin irritation. Gel packs offer a higher level of comfort, but come at a higher potential cost. Although frozen peas are a convenient and inexpensive choice, the cold they give might not be sufficient for some individuals. Ice water baths are incredibly efficient, but they are not always convenient because they take a lot of time.

Cryotherapy chambers are somewhat costly, yet they deliver a stable dose of cold therapy to their users. Cold compression wraps are convenient and easy to transport, but it can be challenging to get them to stay in place. In the end, the technique of cold treatment that will work best for you will be determined by the specific requirements and preferences of your condition.

3. Step 3: Set Up Your Treatment Area

It is essential to prepare your treatment area thoroughly before beginning the cold therapy treatment that you have chosen. During your therapy, this will help you maintain a comfortable and secure state. Check to see that the environment is tidy and devoid of any debris. You are also going to need something to sit on, such as a towel or a mat. If you intend to use ice packs, you need first fill a sink with cold water and then set the ice packs inside the sink. If you are going to use a cold gel pack, make sure that you place it in the freezer at least two hours before your treatment.

4. Step 4: Start Slow with Short Sessions

When beginning cold therapy for the first time, it is essential to progressively extend the amount of time spent undergoing the treatment. To get started, try out several treatments that don't go on for longer than five minutes. You will be able to tolerate longer bouts of cold exposure as your body develops acclimated to the discomfort of the lower temperatures. Because of this, you won't have to worry about experiencing any of the potentially unpleasant side effects, such as pain or shock. In addition, making a modest start will allow you to evaluate how well your body reacts to the cold treatment. Before commencing any therapy, you should see your physician if you suffer from any medical disorders that might be worse by being exposed to frigid temperatures.

5. Step 5: Monitor Your Progress and Adjust as Necessary

The application of cold treatment over a prolonged period produces the best results. However, if you discover that your symptoms are not better after several weeks of treatment, you must talk with your physician to determine whether or not a different course of treatment will be more beneficial for you.

It's possible that adjusting the frequency or length of your treatments might help ease the symptoms you're experiencing.

In addition, your doctor may advise you to participate in various complementary therapies, such as heat therapy, to assist in the reduction of your discomfort. You can make certain that your cold therapy sessions are providing you with the most amount of benefit by keeping track of your progress and modifying your approach as required.

This beginner's guide will assist you in getting started with cold therapy if you are contemplating beginning the treatment. Keep in mind that you should begin your sessions cautiously and progressively extend their duration as your body grows more acclimated to the frigid temperatures. If, after many weeks of therapy, your symptoms have not improved, you must monitor your progress and discuss the matter with your primary care physician.

HEAT THERAPY VS. COLD THERAPY

When it comes to finding relief from pain, a lot of individuals aren't sure if heat therapy or cold therapy is going to be more effective for them. Each approach has some advantages as well as disadvantages. In the end, it comes down to a personal choice that is determined by the nature of the agony that you are in. Let's take a more in-depth look at the benefits and drawbacks of each approach so that you can make an educated choice about which one is the most appropriate for your situation.

Heat Therapy Pros

- Increases blood flow, which can reduce inflammation and stiffness.
- Can relax muscles and relieve tension headaches.
- Draws out impurities and can improve circulation.
- Reduces pain by numbing nerve endings.
- Can be comforting and relaxing.

Heat Therapy Cons

- Can increase inflammation in some cases.
- Improper use can result in burns.
- Can make some pains worse, such as migraines or cluster headaches.

Heat treatment is most effective for treating persistent pain, stiffness, and headaches caused by tension. If you are experiencing severe pain as a result of an accident, it is preferable to apply ice to the affected region for the first forty-eight hours to minimize inflammation. If the pain does not go away, you should move to heat therapy. If you suffer from diabetes or heart disease, you should discuss the use of heat therapy with your physician before beginning treatment. Increased blood flow has the potential to make these diseases worse.

Cold Therapy Pros

- Reduces inflammation by constricting blood vessels.
- Decreases swelling and numbness by numbing nerve applied too intensely
- Decreases muscle spasms by reducing nerve activity
- Provides temporary relief from acute pain.

Cold Therapy Cons

- Can cause local tissue damage if used for too long
- Increases risk of cold injuries if used on bare skin or damp skin.
- Not as effective at alleviating chronic pain.

- May not be tolerated well by people with Raynaud's arthritis.

The acute pain, inflammation, and swelling that are best treated with cold treatment are the first two. Although it is not as efficient at easing chronic pain, it can be good in reducing stiffness and soreness. However, it is not as effective at relieving acute pain. Before beginning this treatment, you should discuss it with your physician if you have a medical condition, such as Raynaud's arthritis, that makes your skin more sensitive to the cold.

The use of heat therapy and cold therapy both have their benefits and drawbacks. Because certain illnesses might be made worse by either heat or cold, you must discuss your treatment options with your physician before using either strategy.

Once you have been permitted to utilize either approach, it is entirely up to you to decide which one you believe will be more successful for you. You should give both of these approaches a go and evaluate which one delivers the most amount of relief for the particular sort of pain you are experiencing.

RISKS OR POTENTIAL SIDE EFFECTS OF COLD THERAPY

Before beginning any new treatment, it is crucial to be informed of all of the possible adverse effects, and cold therapy is not an exception to this rule. The use of cold treatment is generally safe and well tolerated, but there are a few hazards that should be kept in mind.

Skin Damage: Cold treatment, which is frequently used to alleviate pain and reduce swelling, can cause skin damage if the patient is exposed to the cold for an extended period. Because of the lower temperatures, the blood vessels in the skin contract, which increases the risk of tissue injury. In addition, because there is less blood flowing to the region, the skin can become dry and cracked. If your doctor has prescribed cold treatment for you, follow his or her instructions to the letter and take special precautions to prevent causing any harm to your skin.

Frostbite: Cold treatment is frequently used to ease pain and inflammation, but it can also create numbness in the area that's been afflicted by the condition. This is because exposure to cold numbs the nerve endings, which in turn can cause a lack of feeling. In most cases, numbness is just transitory and will go away after the affected area has returned to its normal temperature.

However, if the numbness continues for more than a few minutes, this might be a symptom of frostbite on the affected area. Frostbite is a dangerous ailment that can develop when the skin and tissue of the body are subjected to temperatures that are significantly below freezing. You should seek medical assistance as soon as possible if you think you could have frostbite.

Muscular Cramps: Muscle cramps are brought on by involuntary muscle contractions, which can be brought on by exposure to cold temperatures. Cramps are notoriously uncomfortable and can make it challenging to move the leg that is afflicted. Stop using the ice immediately and get some medical assistance if you start experiencing muscular cramping after undergoing cold treatment. Other things, such as being dehydrated or having an electrolyte balance that's off, might also bring on cramps. To avoid cramping, it is important to take in a sufficient amount of fluids and maintain a nutritionally sound diet.

Fatigue: Fatigue is a typical side effect of many different types of exercise, and it is a condition that can be made worse by being exposed to chilly temperatures. When the human body is subjected to temperatures that are too low, it must waste a tremendous quantity of energy to maintain its normal temperature. As a consequence of this, individuals who are subjected to frigid temperatures for lengthy periods may develop feelings of weariness.

A side effect of cold therapy is weariness since the body will burn a lot of energy attempting to remain warm during the treatment. Having said that, exhaustion is not always a negative thing. A few athletes swear by the effectiveness of cold treatment as a means to improve their overall performance. They will be able to train their bodies to be more resistant to the symptoms of exhaustion if they first put themselves in a state of fatigue. They can maintain a greater level of performance for longer periods as a direct consequence of this.

Headache: Headache is yet another potential adverse consequence of receiving cold treatment. The cold can cause the blood vessels in the head to become constricted, which can result in headaches. In addition, the body's reaction to the cold may be the production of chemicals that are the root cause of headaches. On the other hand, these adverse effects are often moderate and disappear on their own over time. Stop using the cold treatment and see a medical professional if your headaches become more severe or if you suffer any other major adverse effects.

Dizziness: Dizziness is yet another potential adverse effect that might be brought on by cold treatment. Because the cold causes blood vessels in the brain to constrict, someone who is cold may experience symptoms including dizziness or lightheadedness. In addition, dehydration may produce dizziness, and those who are exposed to low temperatures may be more likely to get dehydrated as a result of their exposure to the cold. If you feel faint or lightheaded at any time during or after your cold therapy session, make sure you drink a lot of water, sit down, or lie down until the sensation passes. Contact your physician if you are still experiencing feelings of dizziness or unsteadiness.

Irritation: The cold has the potential to make individuals feel uncomfortable, which can then lead to emotions of irritability or agitation. You must see your physician before beginning cold treatment if you have a history of easily becoming irritated or irritable. Together, you'll be able to determine whether or not the advantages of cold treatment are worth the possible downside of experiencing an increase in irritability.

The use of cold therapy is an excellent method for lowering stress, improving mental acuity, and enhancing physical performance. Nevertheless, therapy of this kind should not be approached flippantly because it does carry some degree of danger. Before undergoing cold treatment for any reason, you should make an appointment with your primary care provider.

During the procedure, pay close attention to how your body responds to it, and if you have any uncomfortable side effects, such as cramping, weariness, headache, dizziness, or discomfort, you should cease using the ice immediately. You may get the benefits of cold treatment if you put in the necessary work to prepare and take the necessary safety measures.

WHO SHOULD NOT USE COLD THERAPY?

The use of cold therapy is an excellent method for lowering stress levels, improving mental function, and enhancing physical prowess. On the other hand, it is essential to be aware of the possible hazards that are involved with cold treatment. The following are some of the conditions that may put you at a greater risk of suffering adverse effects:

People with Raynaud's Disease: Patients who suffer from Raynaud's syndrome should not use cold therapy. A disorder known as Raynaud's syndrome is characterized by blood vessel constriction in reaction to exposure to cold temperatures or emotional strain. This might result in a tingling or numbing sensation in the hands and feet. In extreme circumstances, it can also result in gangrene or sores on the skin.

Patients Who Suffer from Sensitive Skin: Cold therapy, also known as cryotherapy, is a treatment that involves the use of cold temperatures to alleviate discomfort. It is not suggested for persons with sensitive skin, even though it may be useful for certain individuals. This is because exposure to low temperatures can cause blood vessels to contract, which in turn results in decreased circulation and oxygenation of the skin.

Additionally, exposure to cold can cause an inflammatory reaction in the skin, which can manifest as redness, swelling, and itching in the affected area. Because of these factors, it is essential to confer with a medical professional before undergoing cold treatment, particularly if you have very sensitive skin.

People with Certain Mental Health Conditions: People who have certain mental health conditions may be more susceptible to the negative impact that being exposed to cold temperatures may have on a person's body, both physically and mentally. For instance, it might cause a rise in heart rate and blood pressure, as well as shivering and muscular spasms. Additionally, it can cause the muscles to tighten. It is also known to contribute to feelings of anxiety and despair in certain people. It's possible that people with certain mental health issues, such as anxiety and depression, will discover that cold treatment makes their symptoms even more severe.

It is crucial to be informed of the potential hazards before starting any treatment, particularly one that involves the use of cold therapy, which is sometimes used as a treatment for physical ailments. If you suffer from a mental health issue, you should see your physician before deciding whether or not to participate in cold treatment.

People Who Have Diabetes: Diabetics should avoid utilizing cold treatment since it might cause the blood vessels to tighten, which can have serious consequences. This might result in a reduction in the blood supply to the hands and feet, which can make diabetic nerve pain even more severe. In addition, those who have diabetes have a greater likelihood of experiencing frostbite.

The condition known as frostbite takes place when the skin and the tissue just underneath it freezes. The hands, feet, nose, and ears are the body parts that are most frequently affected by it. Because people with diabetes have slower blood circulation and less feeling in their extremities, they are at a greater risk of acquiring frostbite. If you have diabetes and are thinking about utilizing cold treatment, you should make an appointment with your primary care physician first.

People Who Already Have High Blood Pressure: Patients who already have high blood pressure should utilize cold treatment with extreme caution since it has the potential to produce a transient rise in blood pressure. If you already have high blood pressure, you need to make sure that you keep a careful eye on your blood pressure while undergoing cold therapy and that you stop the treatment if you see any kind of rise in your blood pressure.

Patients with Renal Illness: Patients who have kidney disease frequently have a buildup of toxins in their blood, which can result in weariness, muscular pains, and other health issues. The application of cold, whether in the form of ice packs or a cold bath, can help reduce pain and inflammation. Cold treatment, on the other hand, should be avoided by persons who have a renal illness because it might cause the body to reabsorb toxins that have previously been filtered out by the kidneys. People with kidney disease should avoid using cold therapy.

The use of cold treatment can also cause blood vessels to constrict, which can lower the amount of blood flowing to the kidneys and further damage their ability to function. Therefore, those who suffer from renal illness should see their primary care physician before beginning any kind of cold therapy.

People with Heart Disease: People who have heart disease should exercise extreme caution when undergoing cold treatment since it might potentially exacerbate their condition. This is because exposure to cold temperatures can promote constriction of the blood vessels, which can result in a rise in blood pressure. The cold can also cause your heart rate to rise, which can put further pressure on your heart. This can put additional strain on your heart.

In extreme situations, this can even cause a person to have a heart attack or a stroke. Therefore, cold therapy can be an effective technique to relieve discomfort and swelling; however, if you have high blood pressure, it is crucial to consult your doctor before using this treatment.

Pregnant women: Cold therapy, usually referred to as cryotherapy, is a treatment that includes subjecting the body to temperatures that are far lower than normal. Cold therapy is commonly used on pregnant women. It is beneficial in treating a wide range of illnesses and is frequently used to reduce pain and inflammation.

Women who are pregnant, on the other hand, should steer clear of a cold treatment since it might cause the uterus to contract. This can cause labor to start too soon, in addition to other difficulties. Even though cryotherapy is usually believed to be safe for most individuals, expectant mothers are strongly encouraged to discuss the possibility of utilizing this treatment with their primary care provider beforehand.

Children Under the Age of 12: It is not recommended that children under the age of 12 utilize cold treatment since it can cause damage to the skin, including frostbite, as well as other complications. Young children have skin that is thinner and more sensitive than that of adults, which makes them more susceptible to the harmful effects of the cold.

In addition to this, children have a greater surface-to-body ratio than adults, which puts them at a greater risk of frostbite. As a direct consequence of this, they experience a greater rate of heat loss than adults. Because of all of these factors, it is essential to discuss with a medical professional before administering cold treatment to children who are less than 12 years old.

Conclusion

People have access to a wide range of choices when it comes to the management of their pain. Some people find that taking medication helps them feel better, while others choose to try more natural remedies, such as cold treatment. Cryotherapy, which is more often referred to as cold therapy, is a treatment that involves the use of freezing temperatures to alleviate pain and inflammation.

Ice packs are the most popular kind of cold treatment. Each ice pack session should last between 20 and 30 minutes and should be administered to the afflicted region. Others get respite from their symptoms by using specialized equipment that wraps the body in cold water or air or by taking cold showers or baths. Although there is no scientific evidence to show that cold treatment is useful for controlling all forms of pain, many people feel that it is helpful in the management of arthritis, migraines, muscular soreness, and menstrual cramps.

It is vital to utilize cold treatment only as prescribed by a qualified medical practitioner, even if it might potentially give some advantages. An excessive amount of cold treatment can cause significant adverse effects as well as harm to the skin. Therefore, it is extremely important to see a medical professional before beginning any new method of pain treatment.

FAQ About Cold Therapy

1. What is cold therapy?

Cryotherapy, which is more often referred to as cold therapy, is a treatment that involves the use of extremely low temperatures to alleviate pain and inflammation. The therapy is normally administered by the use of a cold pack or an ice bath, and the length of time spent receiving it might vary in length based on the ailment that is being treated.

2. What conditions can cold therapy help to treat?

The application of cold compresses has proven to be an effective treatment for a wide range of ailments, including arthritis, muscular discomfort, injuries, and inflammation.

3. How does cold therapy work?

The use of cold helps to reduce inflammation and discomfort by causing a decrease in the amount of blood that flows to the region that is being treated. The numbing effect that the low temperatures have on the region is another source of comfort that may be gained from them.

4. Is cold therapy safe?

When performed as instructed, cold treatment is completely risk-free for the vast majority of people. However, certain potential side effects might occur as a result of the therapy, including frostbite and damage to the tissues. Before commencing treatment, it is essential to have a conversation with your physician about any dangers that might be involved.

5. How long does a cold therapy treatment last?

The length of time needed for a cold therapy treatment will differ from patient to patient based on the nature of the ailment being treated as well as the individual's reaction to the therapy. Nevertheless, the majority of treatments last anywhere from 15 to 30 minutes.

6. How often should I receive cold therapy treatments?

The individual's reaction to treatment as well as the ailment that is being treated will both play a role in determining how frequently treatments are administered. However, the majority of patients require between two and three doses weekly.

7. What are the side effects of cold therapy?

The irritation of the skin is the negative consequence of cold treatment that happens the most frequently. This is because the skin becomes irritated when it is in touch with ice or a cold pack for an extended period. Headaches, lightheadedness, and nausea are three more adverse effects that might occur. These adverse effects are often not severe and typically disappear on their own after a few minutes. However, if you do have any serious adverse effects, you should immediately seek medical help and cease the medication you are currently receiving.

8. Who should not receive cold therapy?

People who have specific medical disorders, such as Raynaud's disease, heart disease, diabetes, or circulation issues, should not undergo cold treatment since it is not suggested for them. Avoiding cold therapy treatments is also recommended for expectant mothers and children in their early years. Before beginning any kind of treatment, you should talk to your physician if you have any doubts about whether or not you should have a treatment that involves cold therapy.

References

3 of the easiest ways to get started with cold therapy. (n.d.). Neurohacker Collective. Retrieved November 27, 2022, from https://neurohacker.com/3-of-the-easiest-ways-to-get-started-with-cold-therapy.

6 techniques for cold therapy. (n.d.). Retrieved November 27, 2022, from https://www.painscale.com/article/6-techniques-for-cold-therapy.

Cold therapy (Cryotherapy) for pain management—Health encyclopedia—University of rochester medical center. (n.d.). Retrieved November 27, 2022, from https://www.urmc.rochester.edu/encyclopedia/content.aspx?contenttypeid=134&contentid=95.

Cold water therapy: Benefits of cold showers, baths, immersion therapy. (2020, July 8). Healthline. https://www.healthline.com/health/cold-water-therapy.

Pros and cons of using a cold therapy machine. (n.d.). Campbell County Health. Retrieved November 27, 2022, from https://www.cchwyo.org/news/2022/july/pros-and-cons-of-using-a-cold-therapy-machine/.

The strange history of therapeutic hypothermia. (2021, May 11). https://www.medicalnewstoday.com/articles/curiosities-of-medical-history-the-controversy-of-using-cold-as-a-treatment.